ISBN: 978-0-9972084-3-6

Published by Gingerspark Press

ABOUT THE AUTHOR

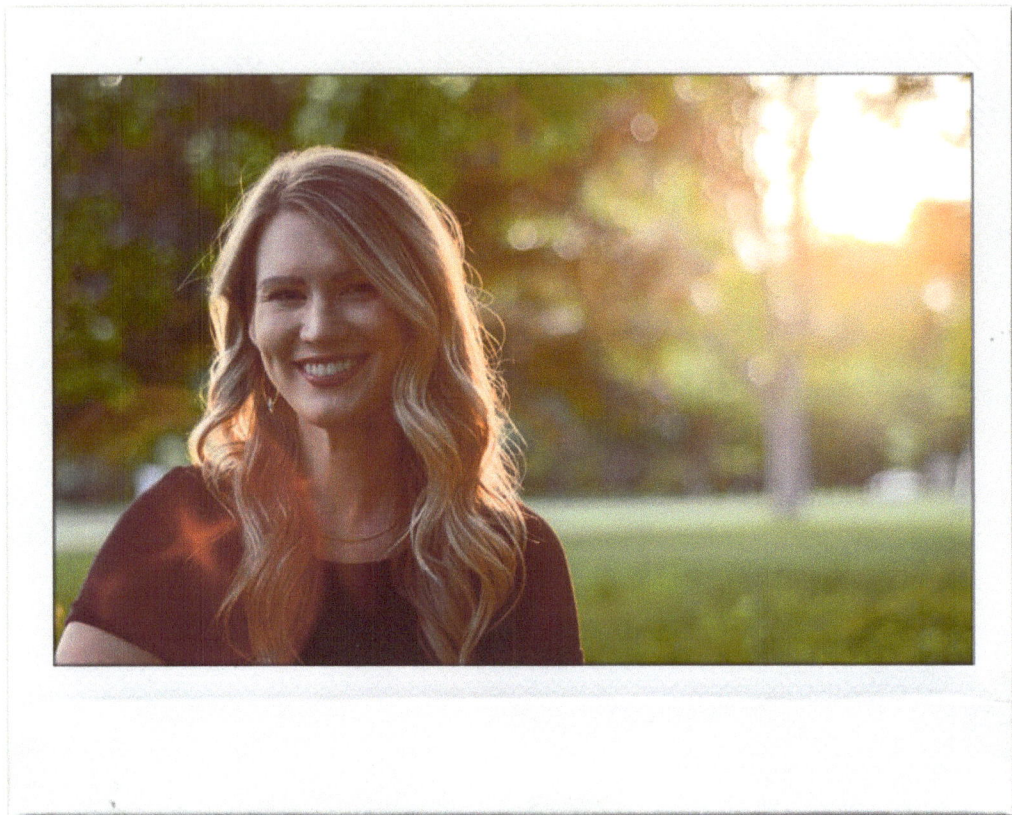

CHRISTIE FREEZE

I grew up a small-town girl, with a very big heart. I spent my childhood on a small ranch in Union, Michigan, raising goats, cows, chickens – you know, all of your typical barnyard friends.

Caring for these animals got me involved with our local 4H Fair, where I served as Club President. Early on, I learned that creating connections was an essential part of how I wished to experience the world – building relationships with incredible people.

I knew that when the time came to build a career, I would want to be in a larger city so I'd have the opportunity to meet even more people and connect with greater networks that inspired growth.

In 2007, I lost my Dad at the age of 46. This experience shifted how I viewed end-of-life planning, aging, and health concerns. It's not always an age-game, and we are not guaranteed any certain amount of years or outcomes. Losing my Dad early on in life has inspired me to live every moment as if it could be the last. Love and compassion are the greatest gifts we can give freely to all whom we encounter.

In 2011, I moved to Indianapolis while in property management, and soon transitioned into Senior Care. I have absolutely loved being in this space for the last 10 years. Early on in the transition, I landed what I endearingly call the "perfect foundation for a senior care profession" at The Stratford, in Carmel, Indiana. The team that surrounded me held a wealth of knowledge that I was eager to absorb. They trained me, taught me the ropes of Senior Care, and as a result, I have gone on to become a trusted resource in our community.

After my time at The Stratford, I went on to help open an Assisted Living Community in Brownsburg, and then transferred to a sister community in Zionsville. These communities had a wider variety of different levels of care and I deeply desired to better understand these systems and how to better connect the average person to the right resources and support while navigating this season of life.

For over a decade now I have helped Family Caregivers like you get connected to the best resource(s) for their exact situation, all while cultivating a self-care practice of their own, maintaining a sense of wellbeing along the way.

Through following my inner voice, I've been guided to trust in the decisions that have led me to establish CAREbyChristie in 2020. It's my greatest intention to equip families (earlier in the process) with the tools and resources needed to navigate caring for an aging loved one, confidently, and with a bit more ease than we have societally experienced in the past.

This is truly my life's work and it's my greatest honor to share this space with you!

xo!
Christie

Roadmap for Eldercare

A Simple Guide Equipping You with Tools and Resources for Eldercare Ease

BY CHRISTIE FREEZE

TABLE OF CONTENTS

ROADMAP FOR ELDERCARE 2.0
MASTER YOUR ENERGY AS YOU NAVIGATE ELDERCARE

WHAT'S INSIDE?

Family Caregivers - The journey often begins at Home and travels down many intricate paths before additional and/or higher levels of care are necessary. We will walk through each piece of the puzzle so that you have a foundation to build upon if faced with something similar.

Healthcare Professionals - Being a quality resource to those you serve is the greatest blessing and you will be far more trusted in your role while stepping into your purpose to serve.

Both - Soul-care is crucial to ease in Eldercare. There are five pages filled with proven practices that are easy to implement, setting you up for maximized energy and effortless ease.

HOW TO USE THIS GUIDE

I recommend flipping through the entire workbook to get an idea of what options are available to you and your family.

WHAT TO EXPECT

My intention with this Roadmap V2.0 is to give you a bird's-eye view of the path most often traveled.

It is of the highest importance that you are equipped with resources that will complement and support your stage and ongoing journey.

Additionally, there are five pages of self-care systems/tools/support to add in, easily.

CAREkey(s) Vocabulary

Adult Day: Daytime relief for caregivers and engaged stimulation for your loved one needing supervision or safety oversight during the day. Great for socialization and purposeful engagement.

Alzheimer's: Disease itself, there are different stages within the disease.

Assisted Living: Neighborhood where assistance with activities of daily living, like bathing, dressing, medication administration 24/7, and nursing staff available. Licensed and unlicensed - know the pros & cons of both!

Continuing Care Retirement Communities (CCRC): All on the same property or under the same roof. Independent living (cottages, separate wing, stand-alone building), assisted living, skilled nursing facilities, and long-term care facilities.

Dementia: Umbrella of symptoms, many different stages and types. (Dementia Friends, Alzheimer's Association)

End of Life Doula: Similar to a midwife, aiming to help families cope with death through recognizing it as a natural and important part of life.

Hospice: A benefit available through medicare/Medicaid that focuses on the patient rather than the disease; maintaining comfort through end of life - best to take advantage of this at time of terminal diagnosis.

Home Care vs. Home Health: Non-medical (companion care/personal service agency) vs. medical care with nursing and licensed medical staff. Home care is typically private pay, but accepting of additional payer sources. Home health is sometimes covered by primary/additional insurances.

Independent/ Retirement Living: Layer of security/amenities to allow independence while allowing relief of day-to-day chores and responsibilities to allow the highest quality of life. Cottage style within continuum of care setting.

Long-Term Care Facilities/ Insurance (LTC): Higher level nursing care, Medicaid accepted, many different options available. There are resources that can review your LTC policy in advance of when you actually want/need to use it to help you prepare based on your wishes and know your options for maximum benefit.

Medicare: Insurance that covers many different resources and solutions.

Medicaid: Federal and state program that helps with costs for individuals with limited income.

Memory Care: Secured neighborhood/environment to ensure the safety of your loved one with memory loss while keeping them active and engaged throughout the day, allowing you to have quality visits as a loved one or friend, rather than always as a caregiver.

Palliative Care: Similar to hospice. Assists in improving quality of life. Recommended to start at time of diagnosis and can support you alongside other treatment solutions.

Respite: Temporary housing; hotel-like. Sometimes with supervised care. Helpful for caregivers during vacation, personal time, medical emergency.

Senior Living: Housing designed for seniors or 55+. Often offering additional amenities to engage/socialize onsite and deliver sense of community while maintaining independence. And/or care being provided to a senior or older adult within their living situation.

Skilled Nursing Facilities (SNF): Most often used for short-term stays, post-hospitalization to continue rehabilitation. Medicare/insurance assists with payment for specific length of time.

Veteran's Aid & Attendance: AKA Wartime Pension, 65+ those who qualify.

OVERVIEW OF CARE OPTIONS

HOME, WITH A PLAN

We will take a deeper dive into ways this is possible in the coming pages - but know that it CAN be done safely!

ASSISTED LIVING

Many options available just within this space alone. This is where more hands-on healthcare support is available in a community-style setting.

SKILLED NURSING FACILITY (SNF)

This is most commonly visited after a surgery or major event, with the intention of rehabbing you back to home. There are occasions where this can become a long-term stay. LTC Insurance/Medicare.

INDEPENDENT/RETIREMENT LIVING

This is a great first step, and often is an incredible lifestyle. The key is to stay open and explore.

MEMORY CARE NEIGHBORHOODS

A great solution for those navigating a cognitive decline and in need of supervised support with a family-style setting.

LONG-TERM CARE (LTC)

Typically where the highest level of care is provided as needs increase. Long-Term Care insurance is something to consider exploring as a payment solution.

HOME, INDEPENDENTLY

SECURITY SYSTEM

HOME MODIFICATIONS

Providing a sense of safety and backup communication method for loved ones in case of emergency.

The options are endless! From furniture risers to supportive devices for added ease.

EMERGENCY PENDANT

HOME CARE/COMPANION SUPPORT

Especially helpful if family/loved ones are out of state or do not live nearby. Alerting help when an accident has occurred can save a life.

This can work in many ways, but is often used to supplement any needs unable to be done by the individual living home alone or when the caregiver needs a break.

FILE OF LIFE/911 CONTACT

Contact me for a free File of Life. You can also get them online or create your own. Basically a cheat-sheet of important emergency information for ambulance, etc., to hang on the fridge.

HOME WITH A LOVED ONE

HOME MODIFICATIONS

The options are endless! From furniture risers to supportive devices for added ease.

ADULT DAY PROGRAMS/ SENIOR CENTER

Provides a sense of safety, socialization and independence for those seeking a like-minded community.

RHEA SERVICES/CAREKIT

There are great options that are available to capture the information needed for emergency ease.

HOME CARE/COMPANION SUPPORT

Provides a sense of safety, support, and backup communication method for families requiring additional hands-on help.

CAREGIVER SUPPORT/RELIEF

There are endless resources for this, the key is finding what works for you, and knowing that may ebb and flow. Stay committed to the practice of exploring what works.

START OPEN CONVERSATIONS

Communicating this type of topic and interest in knowing what your loved ones desire for their path doesn't have to be scary!

Self-Care Basics 101

You are Worthy!

In my experience, this is the biggest reason we don't carve out space for ourselves, feely unworthy of taking the time to do so. Through strengthening our self-trust (intuition), we begin to reclaim our power.

Facts on Caregiver Burnout

According to estimates from the National Alliance for Caregiving, during the past year, 65.7 million Americans (or 29 percent of the adult U.S. adult population involving 31 percent of all U.S. households) served as family caregivers for an ill or disabled relative.

- 84% of caregivers need more help and information with at least 14 specific topics related to caregiving. The top three (3) topics of concern to caregivers are the following:
  - Keeping their loved one safe (42%)
  - Managing their own stress (42%)
  - Making end-of-life decisions (22%)
- Caregivers in high care-burden situations are more likely to seek help (83% versus 73% of low-burden caregivers)

Vibration & Energy

"How we allow ourselves to be fed is a metaphor—if ever there was one—for the vibrational quality of what we're willing to 'take in' that goes well beyond the act of filling our bellies. It's an energetic statement of intent." - Lizzie Shanks

You are capable of creating ease.

We have been taught to dismiss our thoughts and feelings, big and small to get to the next milestone, or even through the day.

Setting our emotions to the side in order to push on or keep going.

It is when we allow ourselves to FEEL all of this in our body, release anything no longer serving us, that we can experience ease and abundance day to day.

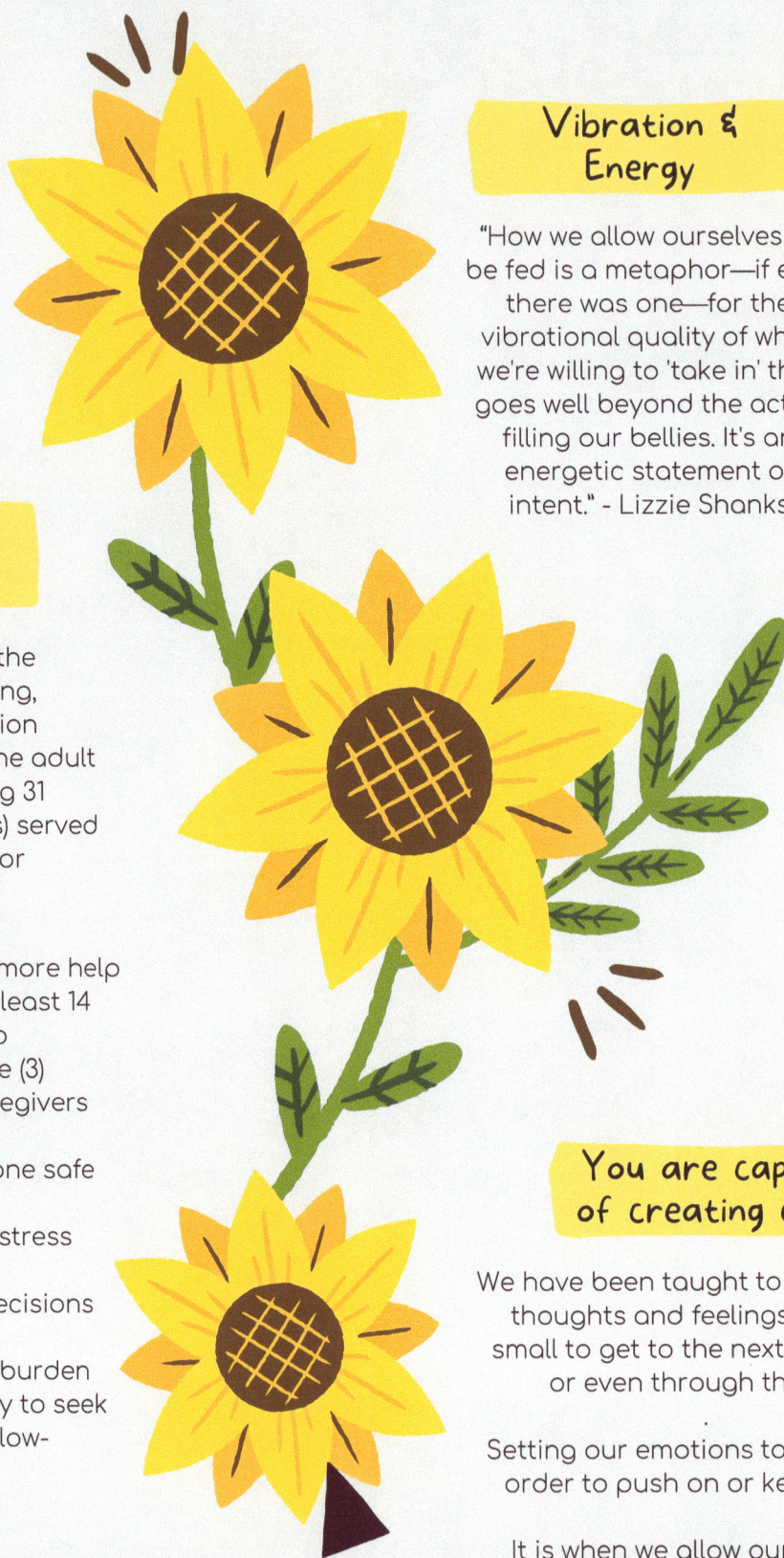

You are safe to create space for yourself ~Christie

HOME MODIFICATIONS

Furniture Risers
Ranging from generic to custom fit, this home modification is an easy first step in adapting your house for safety.

_____

_____

_____

_____

Grab Bar(s)
Many options, sizes, and shapes. The goal is to reach out to them for support proactively, not reactively.

_____

_____

_____

_____

Shower Chair
Showers are the main cause of falls and are generally an unsafe experience if balance is compromised.

_____

_____

_____

_____

Ramps or Stair Chair
This works well for those desiring to remain where they are and are in need of a stair-free experience.

_____

_____

_____

_____

Lift Chair/Bed
Both are game-changers and often can be cozier than the long-time favorite, Lay-Z-Boy.

_____

_____

_____

_____

Assistive Devices
Medication dispensers, video doorbell, camera system, rollator, can, etc.

_____

_____

_____

_____

CAREGIVER RELIEF

Sustainable Self-Care

It is first on this list for a reason: without it, you will experience quicker burnout and exhaustion. Luckily there are a ton of great tools in this roadmap for you!

_____

_____

_____

_____

Adult Day Programs

This allows working and/or busy care partners to continue, while knowing their loved one is safe and having a great time.

_____

_____

_____

_____

Support Group

There is a great value in joining and belonging to a support group. The more connection, the better!

_____

_____

_____

_____

Senior Center

An incredible resource in local communities. A safe location for older adults that engages and stimulates connection daily.

_____

_____

_____

_____

Home Care/Companion

This is helpful when safety and/or isolation is a concern for your loved one and you are the main source of outside connection.

_____

_____

_____

_____

Family Involvement/ Outings with Friends

Crucial to everyone's mental health. There are creative ways to accomplish these visits and outings with ease.

_____

_____

_____

_____

SPOTTING SIGNS FOR ADDITIONAL SUPPORT

1

ISOLATION

Retreating to home more than usual, declining invites to outings, avoiding phone calls.

2

BALANCE/UNSTEADINESS

#1 reason for falls. The domino effect that can occur after a fall can be challenging. Connect with Home Safety Coach to learn tricks and tips.

3

MISSED/MANAGE MEDICATIONS

This is CRITICAL. Resources are available to automate this process if needed.

4

UNOPENED MAIL/UNPAID BILLS

This is something that often gets overlooked. Be sure to not shame or embarrass your loved one, but take note of this clue.

5

DINGS/DENTS IN VEHICLE

Make it a practice to do a quick scan of your loved one's vehicle for any bumps or bruises it may have acquired.

6

WEIGHT LOSS/EXPIRED FOOD

Both should raise a bit of concern. Note this as a red flag.

(Self) Awareness

You are Safe.

Begin to look around your physical reality and see if you can identify what you smell, see, hear, taste, and feel on your skin. This will bring you into the present moment any time you are needing to feel grounded and in your body.

Words are Power

The words we use towards ourselves and others have a greater impact than you may realize.

Our subconscious mind does not know the difference between "joking" or not, and our cellular level retains the harsh or hurtful words we speak.

Track to Attract

Start a Notes thread in your phone, or write in a planner or journal- 10 things each day that you can find to be grateful for. It only takes a couple minutes, and as a result- more things to be grateful for will be attracted into your life.

Practice your way!

Journaling (or any modality) doesn't have to "look" a certain way, find what feels good for you. Notes section of your phone, a dollar store pack of 5, or a journal for each area of your life you are interested in exploring deeper. There is no "wrong" way to do this.

It will continue to evolve, change, and grow!

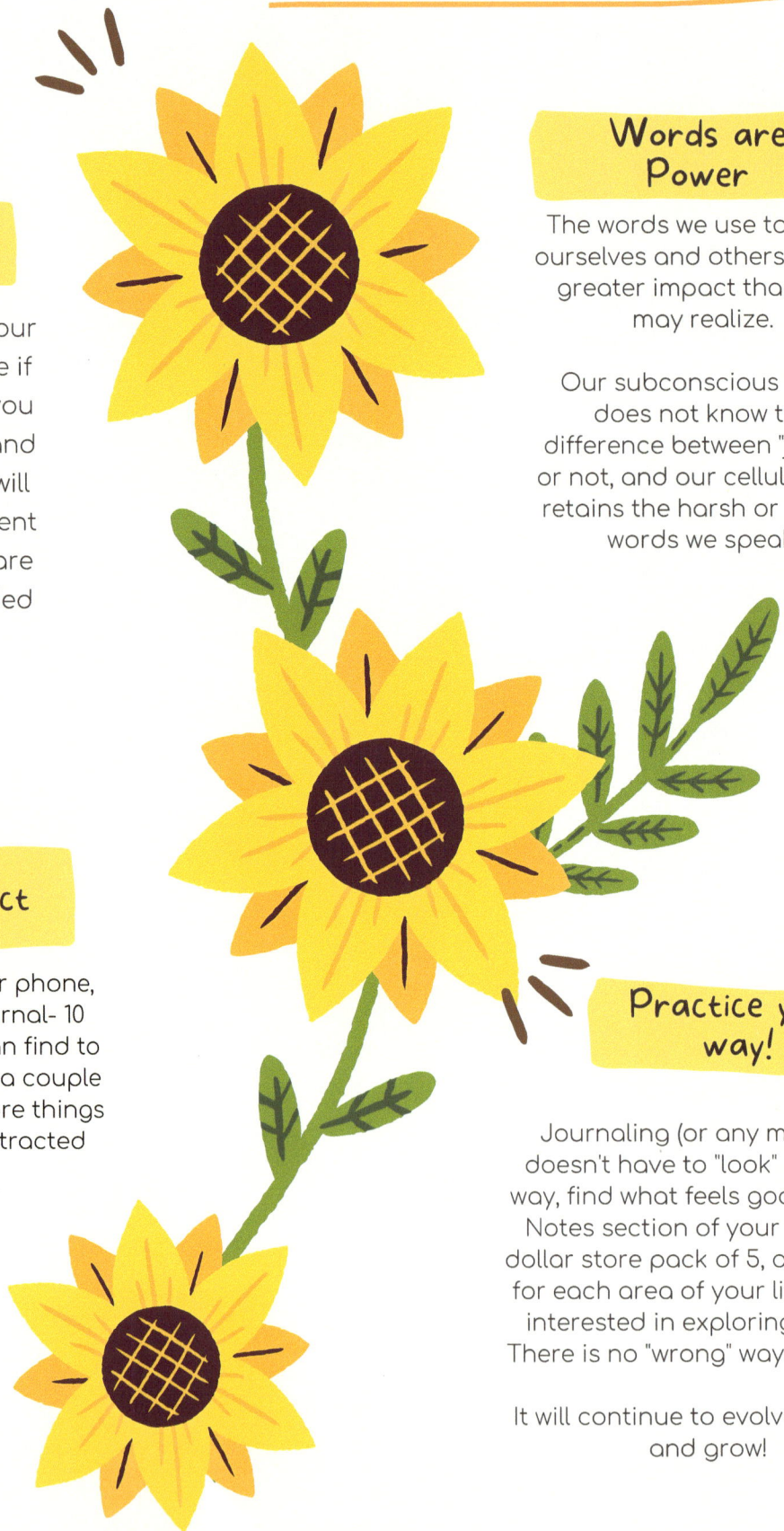

"There are only four kinds of people in the world. Those who have been caregivers. Those who are currently caregivers. Those who will be caregivers, and those who will need a caregiver." — Rosalyn Carter

KEY PLAYERS FOR YOUR CARE JOURNEY

FAMILY CAREGIVER COACH

The Memory Compass is a great resource, along with additional specialties that are available to support your family as you navigate.

ELDER LAW ATTORNEY

There are many ways elder law attorneys can help. Their specialty provides an added layer of resources and support.

FINANCIAL ADVISOR/CPA

Being proactive versus reactive with this resource is key. There are so many benefits and ways to pay for care needs and it's best to discuss them early.

GERIATRIC CARE MANAGER

This is a great resource to keep all care needs in order and communicate effectively between all parties, keeping everyone in the loop.

PHYSICIAN TEAM

Oftentimes the care team is made up of multiple physicians and practitioners. It's important to keep records organized and accessible.

SENIOR LIVING ADVISOR

This is a great resource to navigate your senior living community search. Find who you connect with best and let them guide you.

PREPARING THE VILLAGE

SHARING THIS ROADMAP

Having a foundation of information to build on is key.

GATHERING THE FAMILY PLAYERS

Gather those family members who wish to/should be involved and divvy up tasks based on strengths.

DECISION MILESTONES

Determine and agree upon when to add care or support, higher levels of care, etc.

KNOWING THE WANTS/WANT-NOTS

If you are taking the lead on providing or acquiring additional care, consider asking your loved one (or self) what you do/do not want.

GO-TO BOOK/BINDER/PDF

Complete as fillable pdf with RHEA services or compile all your most important documents into one easy to access location for emergency.

GET STARTED

It truly is never too early to get started and using this guide as your starting point guarantees you are not left to figure it out alone.

ELDER LAW BENEFITS

TRUST/WILL/ESTATE PLAN

SO important! Oftentimes, folks don't think they need to consider this "yet." If you are having that thought, the time is now.

POWER OF ATTORNEY

Proactive vs. reactive is key here and is sometimes divided into Financial and Healthcare POA roles.

MEDICAID

This is becoming a more common method of payment when private pay funds are limited. Many communities and healthcare providers accept this form of payment.

ADVOCATE/GUARDIANSHIP

Important for those who may not be able to advocate for themselves; can be anyone requesting and granted Guardianship.

VETERAN BENEFIT(S)

Often an overlooked benefit and applying can be complicated, but there are amazing resources that specialize in that process.

COMPLIMENTARY CONSULT

Many offer a complimentary meet and greet. Find who you connect with and learn how they can help you.

(Self) Acceptance

You are Radical!

Cultivating Self-Love is a game-changer.
Radical Self Acceptance is a way to love and feel grateful for where you are, right now. Know that everything is working out FOR you, not against you.

Modalities & More

There are so many different options to try!

EFT (Tapping)
Meditation
Yoga
Plant Medicine (CBD)
Massage Therapy
Reiki
Accupuncure
Chiropractic Care

Affirmations

- These can be challenging without the right approach. If you are someone who has affirmations that really resonate- stick with those and repeat them often!

  If you are struggling to believe they are true, try adding "I am choosing to believe _____".
  Ex: "Today I am choosing to believe that I am worthy of ease and capable of caregiving success.

- I recommend downloading the "I Am" app on your phone and allowing the notifications. They are so helpful and an unexpected boost throughout the day! Learning the way in which your subconscious receives affirmations is helpful!
  "I choose, I am becoming, I am learning _____" feels better for those who are averse to the traditional "I AM" statements.

The Compound Effect of MicroPromises.

By mastering Micropromises and strengthening our self trust, we are able to layer in more nurturing practices and space for ourselves, into the day to day experience that we know set us up for success and ease.
Build self trust so that when you come up against an obstacle, you can handle it with more self compassion..

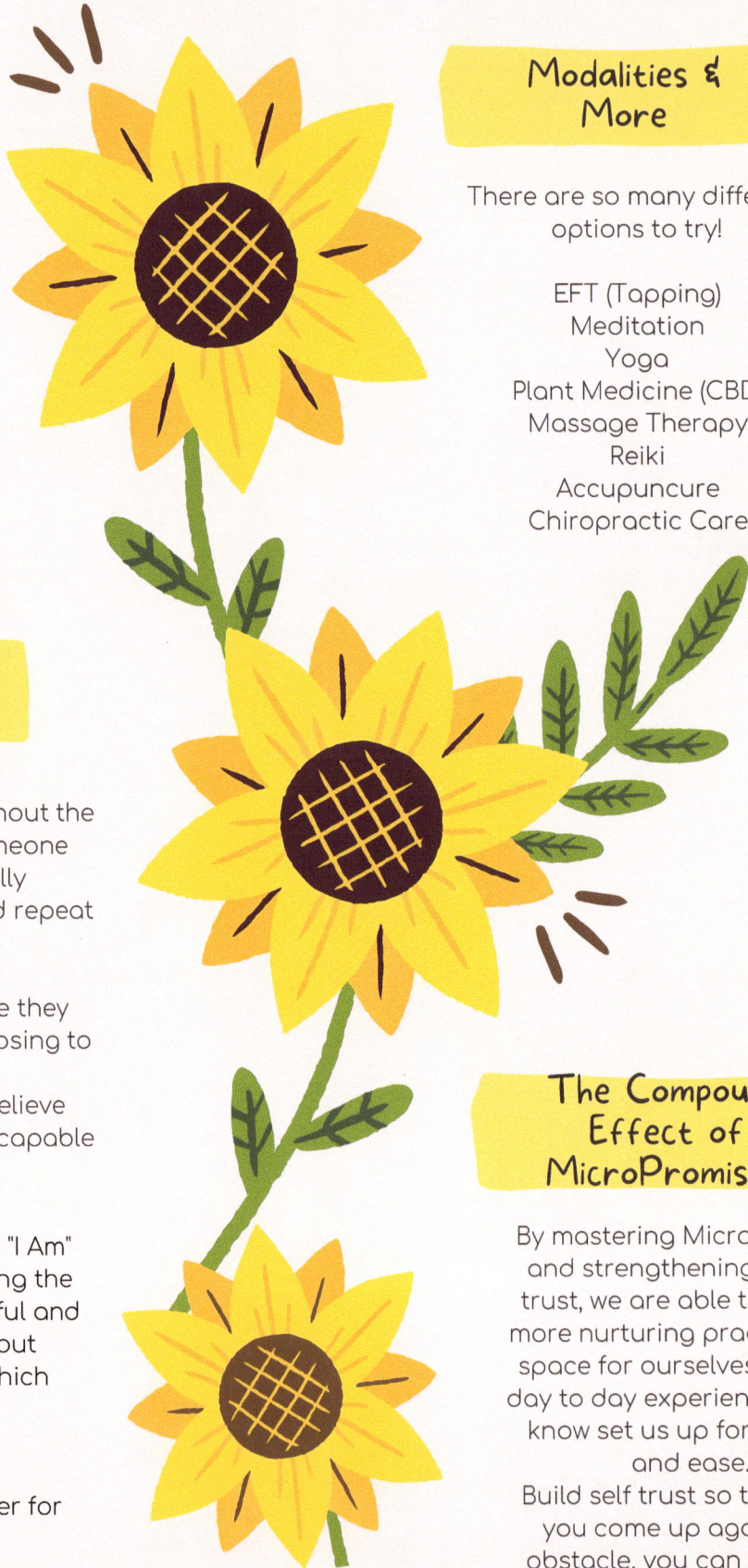

PHYSICIAN OPTIONS

Traditional PCP
Many keep their Primary Care Physician and add specialties as needed.

_____

_____

_____

_____

Mobile/Travel Doctor
Grace At Home and MyMobileMD are local options available.

_____

_____

_____

_____

Case/Care Manager (RN)
Adding a layer of communication and providing families with updated accurate information.

_____

_____

_____

_____

Specialist in Geriatric Care
There is value in a broad care team, chiropractic care + therapists offer many solutions to fill in the gaps of traditional medicine.

_____

_____

_____

_____

Reliable Transportation
Oftentimes why doctor appointments are missed.

_____

_____

_____

_____

Dentist/Podiatrist/Optometrist
Don't forget to visit your routine appointments. Proactive vs. reactive is always our goal.

_____

_____

_____

_____

DRIVING DECISIONS

The Dings/Dents
Scan the vehicle at your visit(s).

_____

_____

_____

_____

Getting Lost
Although this can be frightening, use this as a safety conversation, prompt and implement tools to avoid it happening again.

_____

_____

_____

_____

Driver's Test
This can be requested by a doctor as a routine renewal test. Work with your care team to make this an objective request.

_____

_____

_____

_____

Vehicle Tracker/GPS Device
There are some laws that apply here, but look into what is available for you and explore for a loved one who is driving with a cognitive declline.

_____

_____

_____

_____

Keys
Taking away the keys has been a long-time feared event. There are techniques to make this an experience that upholds the dignity of all.

_____

_____

_____

_____

Alternate Transportation Options
Senior centers offer transportation. There are also companies dedicated to providing safe travel for older adults.

_____

_____

_____

_____

CONSIDERING A COMMUNITY

CONSIDER SUPPORT

There is a free resource available that will walk you through this process.

ATTEND AN EVENT

The key to this one is truly going in with an open mindset and allowing the full experience to be soaked in. Good or bad – give it a true shot!

TRUST YOUR GUT

Really stay present during and after your experience.

RESEARCH

Figure out what is most important to you, then research what location has most of that!

TRY THE FOOD/DINING EXPERIENCE

There are so many amazing dining experiences to be had. Try for yourself to see what you like.

GET EXCITED!

This is a new chapter that is as exciting as the many other times you've taken a leap and tried something new – has it mostly worked out for the best?

MEMORY CARE & SUPPORTIVE SERVICES

ADULT DAY PROGRAMS

Providing community and stimulation for those navigating a cognitive decline, often keeping the individual in high spirits, limiting behaviors.

STAND ALONE MEMORY CARE NEIGHBORHOODS

Increasing in popularity due to their home-like environment, often no more than 8-10 residents per house.

SKILLED MC WITHIN A LTC COMMUNITY

Higher levels of care provided for those needing full-time assistance and advancing needs.

MEMORY CAFÉS

They are offered monthly, allowing families to engage and connect with their loved one in a conducive environment.

ASSISTED LIVING MEMORY CARE

A secure neighborhood that allows for a smooth transition out of traditional AL into MC while maintaining independence and dignity.

DEMENTIA FRIENDS/CICOA/ ALZHEIMER'S ASSOCIATION

The Memory Compass provides dementia family coaching.

DISEASE-SPECIFIC RESOURCES

ALZHEIMER'S/DEMENTIA

01

ALZHEIMER'S ASSOCIATON

800-272-3900
alz.org

02

DEMENTIA DARLING

dementiadarling.com

03

THE MEMORY COMPASS - DEMENTIA FAMILY COACHING

thememorycompass.com

ARTHRITIS

01

ARTHRITIS FOUNDATION

800-283-7800
arthritis.org

02

ACCUPUNCTURE/CHIROPRACTIC CARE

03

ANTI-INFLAMMATORY DIET

PARKINSON'S

01

THE PARKINSON'S FOUNDATION

800-473-4636
parkinson.org

02

SUPPORT GROUPS

03

CLIMB/ROCK STEADY PROGRAMS

Inspired Action

You are always taking action, choose to make it an inspired one!

The Illusion of Time

Oftentimes we feel like we do not have "enough time" to do the things we want or need- and find it hard to prioritize what action step to take, first!

Get clear on what is most important and block off time for just that- watch time expand!

Schedule it in!

- This hack has been a game-changer for many. If you are someone who is fairly confined to the calendar on their phone or attached to yo email- start sending yourself Self-Care Checkpoints throughout the day/week/month and fill them like every other appointment on your schedule!

- Time block as little as 5 minutes, and up to as much as you need- I often will choose one day a month that is a mental-health/recharge day and work daily 5-10 minute practices into the week days!

Brain Dump

A longtime favorite practice and one that has yet to fail me. "Brain-Dump" is where you put everything that is swirling around in your mind -> down on paper.
It doesn't need to look a certain way at this stage- just get it all down. THEN work to prioritize, and devise your inspired action plan based on what seems the most exciting now!

Accountability

Find what feels helpful and encouraging to you!
The FB Group for this Roadmap is a safe place that will continue to grow with support and accountability partners as you navigate your Eldercare role.

"Action is the cure for Fear"
Kathrin Zenkina -

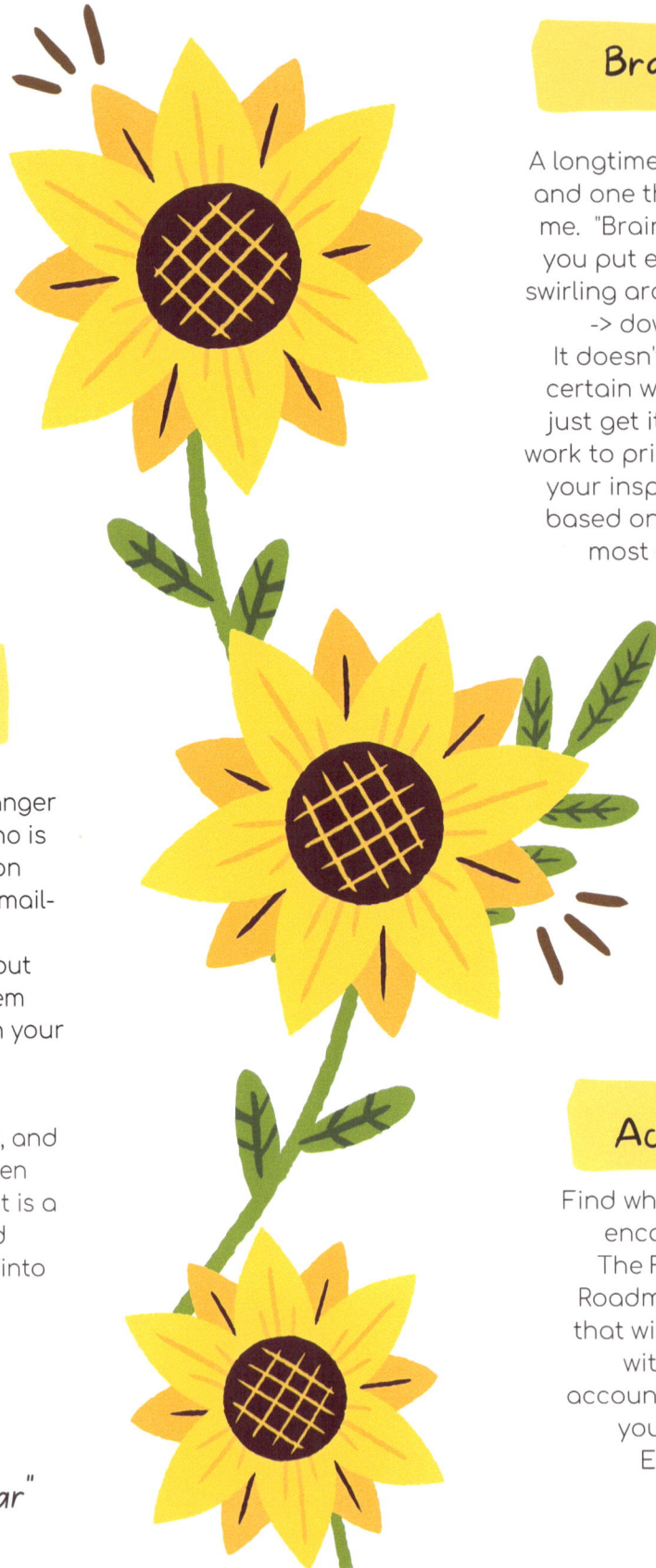

WAYS TO PAY

SALE OF HOME/CONDO

Resources available that specialize in the entire downsizing and sale of home. Senior Real Estate Specialists (SRES) are experienced with this.

LONG-TERM CARE INSURANCE

Important to always be sure to ask about this with your family and loved ones - often it was paid into and forgotten about!

MEDICAID

This is becoming a more common method of payment when private pay funds are limited. Many communities and healthcare providers accept this form of payment.

PRIVATE PAY/INCOME

Some explore using investments, savings, etc.

VETERANS BENEFITS

This is an often overlooked benefit. Applying can be complicated, but there are amazing resources that specialize in that process.

FAMILY SUPPORT

I have seen families do anything from split the costs of care to rotate expenses and offer their inheritance to provide quality end-of-life care.

CELEBRATION OF LIFE

DISCUSS EARLY

There is a free resource available that will walk with you through this process.

HOSPICE BENEFITS

A taboo topic in the aging discussion, but the benefits outweigh the fears associated.

TRUST YOUR GUT

If you feel called to share your Celebration of Life wishes with those close to you, or document them in an easy to access/locate file, do so!

WHAT DO YOU WANT?

Figure out what is most important to you, make sure it's documented, and discussed in a light-hearted way.

END-OF-LIFE-DOULA

A great resource to lean on for additional support in coping with the living and dying experience.

SURRENDER

The path of least resistance is to surrender to the flow of life. You are supported, loved, and taken care of.

BOOK RECOMMENDATIONS

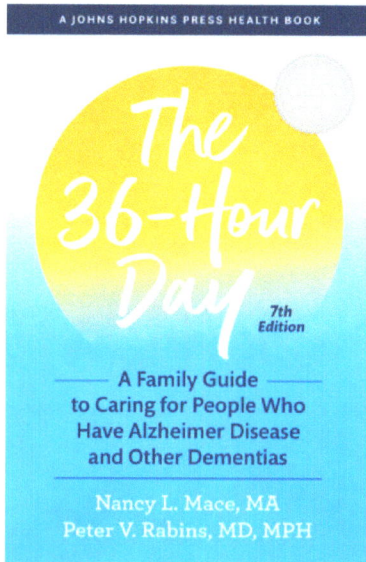

The 36 Hour Day
Nancy L. Mace and Peter V. Rabins

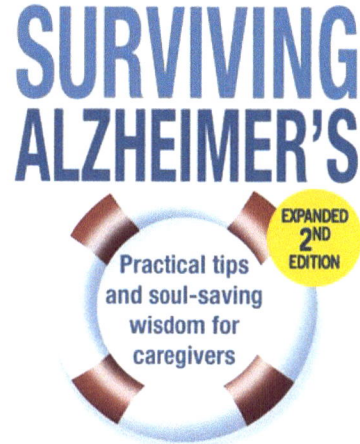

Surviving Alzheimer's
Paula Spencer Scott

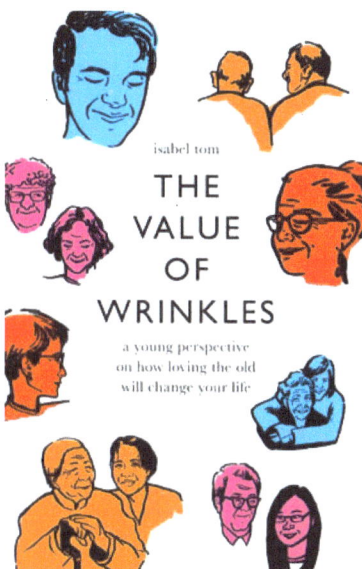

The Value of Wrinkles
Isabel Tom

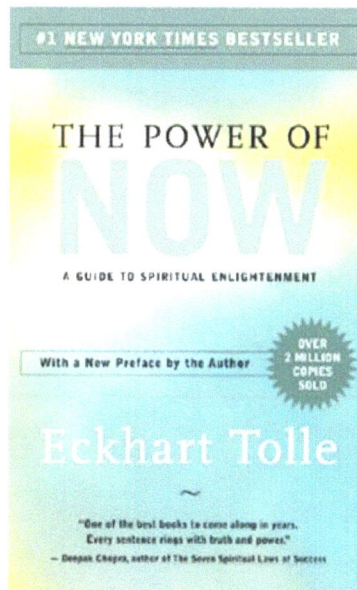

The Power of Now
Eckhart Tolle

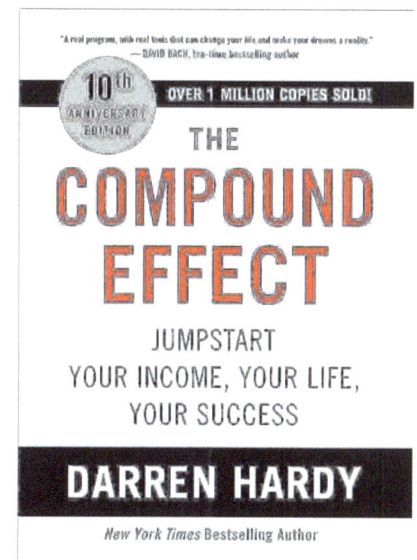

Compound Effect
Darren Hardy

Self-Expansion

You are meant to take up space, and expand!

You are Safe!

By now, I hope you are feeling the self-love begin to cultivate deep within. When you feel safe to take up space and shine your light- that is when you really EXPAND!

Tools to tap into for expansion.

Visualization
Hypnosis
Binaural Beats
Meditation
Tapping
Journaling
Dancing
Creating
Reiki
Movement

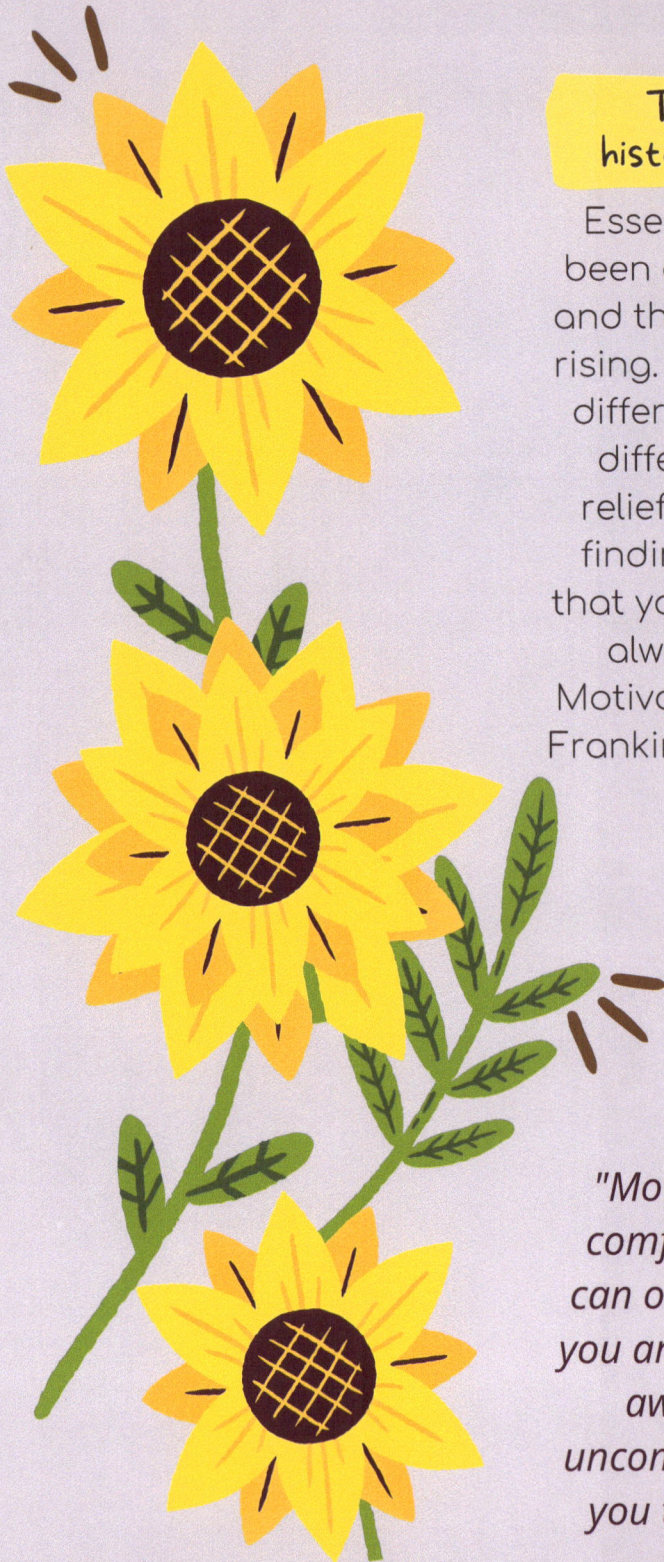

They have a history of healing!

Essential Oils have been around forever, and their popularity is rising. There are many different options for different areas of relief- I recommend finding your Core 4 that you keep with you always. Mine are Motivate/Peppermint/ Frankincense/Copaiba

"Move out of your comfort zone. You can only grow when you are willing to feel awkward and uncomfortable when you try something new.
– BRIAN TRACY

NOTES

NOTES

NOTES

CARE by *Christie*

Uplifting Family Caregivers

Ways to Connect:

- @CAREBYCHRISTIE
- @CAREBYCHRISTIE
- @CAREBYCHRISTIE
- CHRISTIE@CAREBYCHRISTIE
- CAREBYCHRISTIE.COM

www.ingramcontent.com/pod-product-compliance
Lightning Source LLC
Chambersburg PA
CBHW060808270326
41927CB00003B/87